FROM MANAGING TO CONQUERING CORONARY ARTERY DISEASE

Expert Guide To Understanding The Causes, Recognizing Symptoms, And Implementing Effective Treatments For A Heart-Healthy Lifestyle

DR. DASHIELL DANIEL

"From Managing to Conquering Coronary Artery Disease" is an extensive and priceless guidebook that aims to teach readers a deep comprehension of Coronary Artery Disease (CAD), one of the most common and serious cardiovascular disorders. The book, which was painstakingly and meticulously written, goes beyond traditional medical literature in its goal of equipping readers with the knowledge needed to confront and conquer the obstacles presented by CAD.

The early chapters explore the basic concepts of CAD, which lays a solid basis. In addition to extending a cordial greeting to readers, the introduction highlights how vital it is to understand the nuances of this condition. Acknowledging the need for an all-encompassing strategy, the book's goal and parameters are distinctly stated, laying the groundwork for an insightful exploration of the field of computer-aided design.

The first chapter's main topic, "Understanding Coronary Artery Disease," serves as a foundational piece of knowledge. From the definition and etiology of the disease to the discovery of risk factors and diagnostic techniques, it carefully examines all of its aspects. Through a comprehensive examination of the hereditary, behavioral, and medical factors that impact CAD, the book presents a sophisticated picture of the complex nature of this heart disease.

Chapter 2 moves smoothly into a discussion of the many kinds and stages of computer-aided design. The reader obtains a thorough grasp of the range of CAD presentations, from stable angina to myocardial infarction and consequences such persistent complete occlusion and heart failure. The disease's severity is further clarified by means of a methodical grading system.

As the voyage continues, Chapter 3 of the book dives into the topic of treatment strategies, providing insights into both conventional and innovative methods. In order to provide a comprehensive approach to managing CAD, medications, invasive procedures, and novel therapies—such as gene therapy and stem cell treatment—are carefully considered.

In Chapter 4, the emphasis is shifted to lifestyle changes, emphasizing how important healthy behaviors are to preserving heart health. A thorough discussion of diet, exercise, quitting smoking, and stress management is included, highlighting the significance of taking an active role in one's own health.

In Chapter 5, the importance of comprehending the diagnosis, establishing realistic goals, and cultivating productive communication with healthcare practitioners are highlighted, with a strong emphasis on patient education and empowerment. The following chapters cover prevention techniques, integrative heart health approaches, and ways for managing complications related to CAD. The chapters conclude with motivational accounts of individuals who have triumphed over this formidable cardiovascular foe.

All things considered, "From Managing to Conquering Coronary Artery Disease" is an invaluable resource for medical professionals, patients, and everybody interested in learning more about CAD. Empowerment, resilience, and a proactive approach to heart health are encouraged by the book's thorough examination of the condition, available treatments, and lifestyle changes.

Overview

Greetings and welcome to the extensive guide, "From Managing to Conquering Coronary Artery Disease." Coronary Artery Disease (CAD) is a global threat to cardiovascular health, affecting millions of people. With a focus on providing a comprehensive overview of the disease, including its pathophysiology and cutting-edge treatment options, this book seeks to delve deeply into the complexities of CAD. As we set out on this journey, it is critical to recognize the widespread influence that CAD has on world health and the pressing need to create efficient methods of combating this common and potentially fatal illness.

The Value of Knowing About Coronary Artery Disease

Understanding the significant effects of coronary artery disease on cardiovascular health is necessary to completely realize the seriousness of the condition. Heart attacks and other potentially catastrophic outcomes are brought on by coronary artery disease (CAD), which is defined by the narrowing or blockage of coronary arteries, endangering the blood supply to the heart muscle. It is crucial for researchers, the general public, and healthcare professionals to comprehend the complex mechanisms behind CAD. It encourages the development of focused interventions, enables early identification, and gives people the power to make educated lifestyle decisions. Additionally, a thorough understanding of CAD adds to the larger discussion on public health policies by highlighting management and prevention techniques to lessen the burden of this widespread illness.

Goals And Purpose Of The Book

"From Managing to Conquering Coronary Artery Disease" has several goals. First and foremost, it aims to close the knowledge gap between the general public and scientists by offering a resource that demystifies CAD for people with different levels of health literacy.

The book intends to enable readers to actively participate in cardiovascular health promotion and illness prevention by demystifying the complex aspects of CAD. This guide also aims to be a useful resource for medical professionals, providing information on the most recent developments in CAD research, diagnosis, and treatment approaches.

The book's breadth goes beyond traditional debates to include customized therapy, genetic predispositions, and future technology, providing a thorough and innovative approach to overcoming CAD.

The Coronary Artery Disease Pathophysiology

In order to overcome CAD, one must first understand the intricate biology of the disease. Fundamentally, coronary artery disease

(CAD) is caused by the buildup of atherosclerotic plaques in the coronary arteries, which obstruct the heart's blood supply. Atherosclerosis is triggered and worsened by complex interactions between genetic, environmental, and lifestyle factors.

The cellular and molecular processes that lead to plaque development, the function of inflammation, and the effects of risk factors including diabetes, hypertension, and hyperlipidemia will all be covered in this section of the guide.

Through an analysis of the pathophysiological complexities of CAD, readers can acquire significant understanding of prospective therapy targets and preventive measures.

Risk Elements And Preventive Techniques

Comprehending the risk variables linked to CAD is essential for formulating efficacious preventive measures. The guide's section on modifiable and non-modifiable risk factors thoroughly covers everything from age, gender, and family history to dietary habits, level of physical activity, and smoking. The complex interactions between these variables and their combined effects on cardiovascular health will be emphasized.

The handbook will also cover evidence-based preventive strategies, such as pharmaceutical therapies, lifestyle changes, and the application of cutting-edge technologies. Through a thorough examination of risk factors and preventive techniques, readers may take proactive measures to lessen their vulnerability to CAD and strive towards conquering this prevalent cardiovascular disease.

Methods Of Diagnosis And Prompt Identification

The prevention of CAD's severe effects depends heavily on early identification. This section explores the variety of diagnostic modalities that are available, ranging from sophisticated imaging modalities like cardiac computed tomography (CT) and coronary angiography to more conventional techniques like electrocardiography (ECG) and stress testing.

The handbook will clarify the benefits and drawbacks of every diagnostic instrument, highlighting the significance of a customized strategy based on unique patient attributes. Additionally, new technologies and biomarkers that could improve early detection will be investigated.

This guide provides healthcare professionals and the general public with the knowledge required for prompt intervention and improved results by cultivating a thorough awareness of diagnostic approaches.

Innovative Therapies And Approaches

A multifaceted strategy to treatment is necessary to overcome CAD because of the disease's dynamic nature and patient heterogeneity.

This section examines the range of treatment options, from medication and lifestyle modifications to invasive operations like coronary artery bypass grafting (CABG) and percutaneous coronary intervention (PCI). The guide will examine the evidence for each treatment choice, taking into account patient preferences, comorbidities, and the severity of the disease. Furthermore, cutting-edge advancements in the treatment of CAD, such as gene therapy, regenerative medicine, and precision medicine, will be investigated. This guide intends to allow patients and healthcare professionals to make decisions that are well-informed and customized to their specific needs by providing a thorough overview of treatment methods and advances.

Cardiovascular Disease's Psychosocial Aspects

Overcoming the physiological elements of CAD necessitates investigating the psychological factors that impact the course and results of the disease. This portion of the manual will examine how psychological elements like stress, anxiety, and depression affect CAD. It will examine the reciprocal relationship that exists between cardiovascular health and mental health, clarifying the ways in which psychological health might affect treatment adherence, lifestyle decisions, and overall prognosis.

The handbook will also go over how to incorporate psychological therapies into the all-inclusive care of people with CAD, emphasizing the importance of cooperative healthcare teams in meeting patients' needs on all fronts. Both individuals and healthcare professionals can improve the efficacy of treatment approaches and advance long-term cardiovascular health by acknowledging and addressing the psychological aspects of CAD.

"From Managing to Conquering Coronary Artery Disease" seeks to lead the way in empowering people to combat this widespread cardiovascular condition. This guide gives readers the knowledge they need to make wise decisions and actively contribute to the battle against CAD by thoroughly examining the pathophysiology, risk factors, diagnostic techniques, treatment options, and psychosocial aspects of the illness.

The combined efforts of researchers, governments, healthcare professionals, and individuals can pave the way for a future when CAD is not only controlled but conquered as we navigate the complex terrain of CAD.

CHAPTER ONE
A COMPREHENSIVE GLOBAL EXAMINATION

Atherosclerotic plaque buildup in the coronary arteries is the hallmark of Coronary Artery Disease (CAD), a common and possibly fatal cardiovascular ailment. When these essential blood veins are damaged, it can result in a number of problems, such as angina, myocardial infarction (heart attack), and heart failure. These vessels provide the heart muscle with oxygen and nutrition. A mix of lifestyle choices, underlying medical disorders, and genetic predispositions might contribute to the gradual development of CAD.

Reasons And Danger Elements

The development of CAD is significantly influenced by genetics. Because certain hereditary variables can contribute to the production of arterial plaques and a propensity to atherosclerosis, those who have a family history of heart disease are more vulnerable. Finding those who may be genetically prone to CAD requires an understanding of how hereditary genes and environmental factors interact.

A significant influence is also played by lifestyle variables in the development and course of CAD. Risk factors include obesity, high blood pressure, and high cholesterol are developed as a result of sedentary lifestyles, bad eating habits, smoking, and excessive alcohol use. Making lifestyle changes to address these modifiable risk factors is essential to managing and preventing CAD.

Additional factors that contribute to coronary artery disease (CAD) include metabolic syndrome, diabetes, and hypertension. In addition to aggravating existing risk factors, these disorders can encourage atherosclerosis. Controlling these underlying medical conditions is crucial to stopping the advancement of CAD and lowering the risk of unfavorable cardiovascular events.

Signs And Prognosis

Angina, or tightness in the chest, weariness, shortness of breath, and, in extreme situations, heart attacks are common symptoms of coronary artery disease (CAD). Individuals may exhibit different symptoms, and some may not show any signs at all until the disease has advanced enough. Early intervention and successful management depend on the ability to recognize these indicators.

To determine the severity of CAD and to establish its presence, diagnostic procedures are necessary. Non-invasive diagnostic procedures like stress tests and electrocardiograms (ECGs or EKGs) can reveal important details about the health of the heart and possible ischemia. In-depth images of the coronary arteries are provided by advanced imaging techniques such as computed tomography angiography (CTA) and coronary angiography (CAG), which help identify arterial blockages and the need for intervention.

In conclusion, realizing the interaction of hereditary, lifestyle, and medical factors in the development of Coronary Artery Disease is crucial to comprehending the complex nature of the condition. Timely intervention and good care depend on early recognition through symptom awareness and diagnostic techniques.

<u>Overcoming Coronary Artery Disease: Preventive and Therapeutic Approaches</u>

A comprehensive strategy that tackles the underlying causes and risk factors of Coronary Artery Disease (CAD) is necessary for both prevention and management of the condition. For people at risk of or already diagnosed with CAD, a mix of pharmaceutical therapies, lifestyle changes, and, in certain situations, invasive procedures is used to obtain the best possible results.

Making lifestyle changes is essential for CAD prevention. Maintaining a healthy weight and controlling cholesterol levels can be achieved by implementing a heart-healthy diet high in fruits, vegetables, whole grains, and lean proteins. Another essential component is regular physical activity, which lowers the risk of obesity, hypertension, and diabetes while enhancing cardiovascular fitness. In order to reduce the risk of CAD, quitting smoking and consuming alcohol in moderation are crucial.

In order to manage CAD and the risk factors that are linked to it, pharmacological therapies are essential. Prescription drugs like beta-blockers, statins, and antiplatelet medicines are frequently given to treat hypertension, lower cholesterol, and stop blood clots from forming. For people with diabetes, regulating blood sugar levels and adopting healthy lifestyle practices are essential in lowering the risk of complications from CAD.

For those with substantial arterial blockages, invasive operations like coronary artery bypass grafting (CABG) or angioplasty with stent implantation may be advised. By restoring blood flow to the heart muscle, these therapies hope to relieve symptoms and lower the risk of heart attacks. The degree of artery blockages, the patient's general health, and the severity of CAD all play a role in the choice to proceed with invasive operations.

In addition, continuous monitoring and risk factor reduction are part of CAD management. Scheduling routine follow-up sessions with healthcare providers enables the evaluation of treatment efficacy and necessary modifications. For cardiovascular health to remain at its best, blood pressure, blood sugar, and cholesterol levels must all be closely monitored.

A key element of managing CAD is patient education, which provides patients with the information and abilities to take an active role in their care. People can actively manage their cardiovascular health if they recognize the significance of medication adherence, lifestyle changes, and the indicators of deteriorating symptoms.

treating Coronary Artery Disease requires a multimodal strategy that includes pharmaceutical therapies, lifestyle changes, and, if needed, invasive procedures. Through the management of the underlying causes and risk factors, people can lower their chance of developing CAD and enhance their cardiovascular health in general. The long-term therapy of this common cardiovascular ailment requires constant monitoring and patient education.

CHAPTER TWO
TYPES AND STAGES OF CORONARY ARTERY DISEASE

The term "coronary artery disease" (CAD) refers to a group of heart diseases that result from the buildup of atherosclerotic plaques in the coronary arteries. Comprehending the various forms and phases of CAD is essential for efficient handling and averting difficulties.

Stable Angina: A common sign of CAD, stable angina is usually caused by an imbalance in the supply and demand of oxygen in the heart. Stable angina patients have consistent chest pain or discomfort when they exert themselves physically, are under stress, or are in other circumstances that put more strain on their hearts. Rest and nitro-glycerine are common ways to ease this pain.

A partial blockage of the coronary arteries that permits some blood flow to the heart muscle is indicated by stable angina. Changes in lifestyle, medicine, and sometimes revascularization operations such as coronary artery bypass grafting (CABG) are used as management treatments for stable angina.

Unstable Angina: This more concerning form of CAD is characterized by chest pain that does not go away with rest or nitroglycerin and that strikes during rest or with little effort. In contrast to stable angina, unstable angina implies a significant decrease in coronary blood flow as a result of an atherosclerotic plaque rupturing and a blood clot forming. In order to stop the progression of unstable angina to myocardial infarction, it is necessary to take urgent medical action. Anticoagulants, antiplatelet drugs, and coronary angiography are used in treatment to find and treat the underlying lesion causing the problem.

Heart Attack (Myocardial Infarction): The most serious stage of coronary artery disease (CAD) is referred to as a heart attack. It happens when a coronary artery is totally stopped, which causes a section of the heart muscle to die irreversibly from a shortage of oxygen. Severe dyspnea and severe dyspnea are part of the clinical presentation, which may also include nausea and diaphoresis. Minimizing myocardial damage requires rapid reperfusion therapy, which can be achieved with thrombolytic medications or percutaneous cardiac intervention (PCI). In order to stop additional cardiac episodes, post-infarction therapy includes taking drugs such as beta-blockers and ACE inhibitors as well as changing one's lifestyle.

Chronic entire Occlusion: A long-term, entire blockage of a coronary artery is referred to as chronic total occlusion (CTO). CTOs develop gradually as opposed to the abrupt occlusions seen in myocardial infarction. These difficult lesions may restrict available treatments and are a common cause of refractory angina. Even with the development of sophisticated methods and specialized tools, percutaneous coronary intervention (PCI) for CTOs is still a technically challenging procedure for effective revascularization. Coronary artery bypass grafting, or CABG, may be beneficial in certain circumstances for individuals with CTOs in order to restore blood flow to the ischemic myocardium.

Heart Failure and Other Complications: Heart failure is a disorder where the heart's capacity to pump blood is impaired. Coronary artery disease is a contributing factor in this condition. The cardiac muscle may deteriorate as a result of persistent ischemia or infarction as CAD advances. Fluid retention, exhaustion, and shortness of breath are symptoms of heart failure. A higher risk of sudden cardiac mortality, valve anomalies, and arrhythmias are additional complications of CAD. Medication such as beta-blockers, ACE inhibitors, and diuretics are part of the management, as are lifestyle changes and, in certain situations, more sophisticated interventions such implanted devices.

Grading Coronary Artery Disease Severity: A number of grading methods that take into account imaging, angiographic, and clinical factors are frequently used to evaluate the severity of CAD. Among the instruments used to assess the intricacy of coronary lesions are the Syntax Score and the Coronary Artery Surgery Study (CASS) classification. Whether the course of treatment is medical management, percutaneous coronary intervention (PCI), or coronary artery bypass grafting (CABG), these grading systems help clinicians choose the best course of action. In order to customize interventions to each patient's unique needs, grading severity is essential. Variables including lesion characteristics, general health, and patient preferences are taken into account.

clinicians working in the fields of prevention, diagnosis, and treatment of coronary artery disease must possess a thorough awareness of the many forms and stages of the problem. Personalized therapies that are tailored to the unique features of each patient's CAD are crucial to maximizing results and enhancing the general prognosis of those impacted by this intricate and complicated illness.

CHAPTER 3:
CONVENTIONAL AND NOVEL APPROACHES TO TREATMENT

The large burden of cardiovascular illness and mortality is a result of Coronary Artery Disease (CAD), which represents a serious danger to world health. Treating this complicated illness need a thorough understanding of both conventional and cutting-edge therapeutic modalities. When it comes to drugs, antiplatelet medicines are essential for the treatment of CAD. Aspirin and clopidogrel are two examples of medications that impede platelet aggregation, lowering the risk of thrombus development and eventual myocardial infarction. Another mainstay of CAD pharmacotherapy, statins target dyslipidemia by preventing the synthesis of cholesterol, which reduces the development of atherosclerotic plaque. Furthermore, beta-blockers, such as carvedilol and metoprolol, are used to lower blood pressure and heart rate in CAD patients.

This lessens the strain on the heart and increases its effectiveness.

One important aspect of managing CAD is invasive treatments, which provide interventions when medication is not enough. Stent insertion and angioplasty are commonly used procedures to treat clogged coronary arteries. A catheter containing a deflated balloon is inserted into the stenosis location during an angioplasty procedure. The balloon is subsequently inflated, squeezing the plaque and expanding the channel. The next step is to implant a stent, which offers structural support to stop restenosis. A more involved surgical procedure called Coronary Artery Bypass Grafting (CABG) involves rerouting blood around blocked vessels using grafts from other body areas such the internal mammary artery or saphenous vein.

This treatment is especially helpful in cases where more than one coronary artery is impacted.

The field of CAD treatment is always changing as new treatments become available and research continues to uncover new strategies. One possible approach is gene therapy, which aims to treat the genetic basis of CAD. Through the manipulation of gene expression, researchers hope to influence factors that lead to atherosclerosis and improve arterial health. Another innovative method is stem cell therapy, which investigates the ability of stem cells to regenerate damaged heart tissue. By promoting tissue regeneration, this therapy may be able to reverse the course of CAD in addition to lessening its effects.

Antiplatelet medications, such clopidogrel and aspirin, are essential to the treatment of CAD. By preventing platelet aggregation, aspirin lowers the possibility that thrombus will form in coronary arteries.

A thienopyridine derivative called clopidogrel further worsens the prothrombotic environment in CAD by interfering with platelet function through the inhibition of adenosine diphosphate receptors. These drugs are essential for preventing acute cardiovascular events, especially in people who have had a myocardial infarction in the past or who are at a higher risk because of underlying atherosclerosis.

A key component of the pharmacological treatment of CAD is the class of lipid-lowering medications known as statins. These medications, which include simvastatin and atorvastatin, work by preventing the important enzyme 3-hydroxy-3-methylglutaryl coenzyme A (HMG-CoA) reductase from doing its job. Statins slow the development of atherosclerotic plaques and stabilize pre-existing lesions by lowering the amount of low-density lipoprotein cholesterol (LDL-C) in the blood. Statins also have anti-inflammatory properties and enhance endothelial function, which adds to their many advantages in the treatment of coronary artery disease (CAD).

Metoprolol and carvedilol are examples of beta-blockers, which are an essential pharmacotherapeutic choice in the management of CAD. These substances work by blocking beta-adrenergic receptors, which lowers blood pressure, heart rate, and myocardial contractility. Beta-blockers reduce ischemia stress on the myocardium by reducing the cardiac workload; this is why they are very helpful in treating angina and heart failure linked to coronary artery disease (CAD). These medications also have antiarrhythmic qualities, which increases their usefulness in the overall treatment of CAD.

One important component of CAD treatment is invasive treatments, which provide real remedies in cases where conservative approaches are insufficient. Using a catheter with a deflated balloon, angioplasties, which are often carried out by percutaneous coronary intervention (PCI), widen constricted coronary arteries. By compressing atherosclerotic plaque, the balloon expands the lumen of the vessel and allows blood flow to be restored. Angioplasty is frequently followed by the implantation of a stent, which offers structural support to preserve vessel patency. This strategy has been improved using drug-eluting stents, which are coated with drugs that prevent restenosis and so enhance long-term outcomes for patients with CAD.

The gold standard surgical treatment for severe cases of CAD is coronary artery bypass grafting (CABG), particularly in cases when more than one coronary artery is impacted. In CABG, a surgeon makes new conduits to bypass clogged coronary arteries by harvesting grafts, usually from the internal mammary artery or saphenous vein. Through the rerouting of blood flow, CABG helps to improve overall cardiac performance and relieve ischemia symptoms by restoring appropriate perfusion to the myocardium. This treatment is especially helpful for people who have severe coronary artery disease since it offers a long-lasting and all-encompassing solution to difficult anatomical problems.

With the incorporation of new treatments and continuing research, the field of CAD treatment is changing. As a ground-breaking strategy to address the genetic causes of CAD, gene therapy shows promise. The goal is to alter the molecular course of disease by modifying the expression of particular genes linked to vascular inflammation and atherosclerosis. In people with genetic predispositions, this tailored intervention may be able to prevent the onset of CAD in addition to reducing the burden of the illness when present.

Another area of CAD research that is being explored is stem cell therapy, which uses stem cells' capacity for regrowth to heal damaged heart tissue. The potential of several stem cell types, such as induced pluripotent stem cells and mesenchymal stem cells, to encourage tissue regeneration and functional recovery in the ischemic heart is being studied.

According to preliminary research, stem cell therapy may help CAD patients' hearts heal, become more neovascularized, and have better heart function. To clarify the best cell types, distribution strategies, and long-term effectiveness of this novel strategy, more research is necessary.

To sum up, beating Coronary Artery Disease necessitates a multimodal strategy that includes both cutting-edge and conventional treatment options. Pharmacotherapy is based mostly on medications, which target important factors such cardiac workload, lipid metabolism, and platelet aggregation. Examples of these medications are beta-blockers, statins, and antiplatelet medicines. For anatomically difficult cases, invasive procedures like coronary artery bypass grafting and angioplasty provide real answers.

On the other hand, cutting edge treatments such as stem cell therapy and gene therapy represent the vanguard of research and have the potential to fundamentally change our understanding of and approach to treating CAD.

The ongoing integration of these various approaches highlights the dynamic nature of managing CAD, with the goal of addressing the underlying pathophysiology in addition to symptom relief and promoting long-term cardiovascular health.

CHAPTER FOUR
CHANGES TO YOUR LIFESTYLE FOR A HEALTHY LIFE

Reversing coronary artery disease (CAD) necessitates a multifaceted strategy that includes lifestyle changes to support heart health.

This section will cover a wide range of topics, including the need of making lifestyle changes, the benefits of heart-healthy diets like the DASH and Mediterranean, the necessity of regular physical activity and exercise, including strength training and cardiovascular exercise, the necessity of quitting smoking, and the part stress management and mental health play in preventing and treating CAD.

1. The Value of Modifying One's Lifestyle

Making lifestyle changes is essential for managing and preventing coronary artery disease. Living a heart-healthy lifestyle can have a major impact on the cardiovascular health of people with or at risk for CAD. This covers issues with stress management, physical activity levels, tobacco usage, and food choices. Numerous studies have shown that modifying one's lifestyle can help lower the risk factors for coronary artery disease (CAD), including obesity, hypertension, and hyperlipidemia. Adopting a comprehensive strategy for lifestyle adjustments becomes a pillar in the fight against CAD and is a vital adjunct to medicinal therapies.

2. Heart-Healthy Dietary Practices

A key factor in the onset and course of coronary artery disease is diet. Maintaining and avoiding CAD can be greatly aided by eating a heart-healthy diet. The possible cardiovascular benefits of the Mediterranean Diet, which is well-known for emphasizing fruits, vegetables, whole grains, and olive oil, have drawn attention. This diet, which is high in antioxidants and omega-3 fatty acids, has been linked to a decreased incidence of CAD and its risk factors. In a similar vein, the Dietary Approaches to Stop Hypertension (DASH) Diet, which lowers blood pressure, limits sodium intake and includes foods high in nutrients. For those looking to reduce their risk factors for CAD and maximize their nutritional choices, it is essential to comprehend the underlying concepts of these diets.

3. Consistent Physical Activity and Exercise

An essential component of managing and preventing coronary artery disease is physical activity. Frequent exercise has many advantages, such as better weight management, increased insulin sensitivity, and cardiovascular performance. Cardiovascular exercise strengthens the heart muscle and improves blood circulation. Examples of this type of exercise include jogging, swimming, and brisk walking. Strength training activities also complement each other by improving metabolism and total muscle strength.

A comprehensive exercise program that is customized to each person's needs and skills must be followed in order to achieve the best possible heart health.

4. Quitting Smoking

A non-negotiable element of the fight against coronary artery disease is quitting smoking. Smoking has been shown to have negative impacts on cardiovascular health, and it is one of the main risk factors for coronary artery disease (CAD).

Tobacco smoke contains substances that harm blood vessels and aid in the development of atherosclerotic plaques. Giving up smoking lowers the risk of coronary artery disease (CAD) and enhances cardiovascular health in general.

In order to help people, stop smoking, behavioral therapies, medication, and smoking cessation programs are essential. This highlights the significance of a multidisciplinary approach in the fight against CAD.

5. Stress Reduction and Mental Health

Coronary artery disease has been linked to the onset and aggravation of stress, both acute and chronic.

For the purpose of creating successful CAD preventive methods, it is essential to comprehend the complex relationship that exists between stress and cardiovascular health. Stress-reduction methods include mindfulness, meditation, and relaxation training help improve mental health and lessen the body's reactions that cause CAD. Furthermore, treating underlying mental health issues including depression and anxiety is essential to the overall care of CAD. A comprehensive strategy that takes into account a person's physical and mental health is necessary for those managing the complications of coronary artery disease.

beating coronary artery disease requires a multimodal strategy that goes beyond prescription drugs.

A good diet, consistent exercise, quitting smoking, stress reduction, and other lifestyle changes are essential to both preventing and treating CAD. Giving people the information and resources, they need to make wise lifestyle decisions is essential to the continuous fight against this common cardiovascular ailment. These lifestyle modifications have a cumulative effect that improves longevity and well-being by addressing certain risk factors as well as fostering a culture of heart health in general.

CHAPTER FIVE
EDUCATION AND EMPOWERMENT OF PATIENTS
Comprehending Your Medical Diagnose

Patient education is essential to beating coronary artery disease (CAD), beginning with a thorough comprehension of the diagnosis. Patients need to be well-informed about CAD, including its pathophysiology, etiology, and effects on cardiovascular health. This entails explaining the finer points of atherosclerosis, the primary cause of CAD, and how it results in the constriction of coronary arteries, which in turn restricts the amount of blood that can reach the heart.

Patients should also understand the importance of risk factors in the onset and course of CAD, including as hypertension, hyperlipidemia, and lifestyle decisions. Equipped with this understanding, people can make well-informed choices regarding their well-being, contributing to the avoidance and control of CAD.

Establishing Reasonable Goals

In order to overcome CAD, patients must be able to take an active role in their own therapy by setting reasonable goals. These objectives could include changing one's way of living to include things like eating a heart-healthy diet, exercising frequently, and giving up smoking. Setting goals includes managing stress, adhering to drug regimens, and scheduling routine medical examinations in addition to lifestyle modifications. It is essential to customize these objectives to the particular circumstances of every patient, making sure they are both reachable and long-lasting. In order to support patients through this process and create a collaborative environment that encourages patient autonomy and motivation, clinicians are essential.

Adherence To Medication

Medication adherence, in which patients regularly adhere to prescribed drug regimens, is a crucial part of CAD care. A thorough grasp of the recommended drugs, including their methods of action, potential side effects, and the significance of adherence, is necessary to achieve the best possible outcomes in the battle against CAD. Healthcare professionals should have a thorough discussion with patients, clearing up any doubts and worries that can prevent them from adhering to a treatment plan. It is essential to highlight the long-term advantages and the part that drugs play in averting severe cardiovascular events. Furthermore, it is recommended that healthcare institutions incorporate tactics like prescription reminders, educational initiatives, and routine follow-ups to facilitate patients' successful adherence to prescribed medication regimens.

Keeping An Eye On Your Health

Keeping an eye on one's health is a proactive approach to conquering CAD, combining professional and self-evaluation. Patients should be trained to identify signs of CAD aggravation, such as weariness, shortness of breath, and chest pain. Monitoring blood pressure, cholesterol, and blood glucose levels on a regular basis is essential for evaluating the effectiveness of treatment and the progression of the condition. Patients who participate in self-monitoring are better equipped to keep an eye on their health and take immediate action when needed. In turn, healthcare professionals are essential in helping patients learn how and when to self-monitor, which promotes a team approach to CAD treatment.

Interacting with Healthcare Professionals:

Conquering CAD requires effective communication between patients and healthcare professionals.

Patients must be at ease addressing lifestyle obstacles, reporting symptoms, and voicing concerns.

Conversely, healthcare professionals should encourage candid communication by paying close attention to what patients have to say and answering all of their questions. Treatment plans should also be communicated clearly to patients so that they are actively involved in joint decision-making and can comprehend the reasoning for interventions. A continuous feedback loop is created by routine follow-up visits and health education programs, which allows for management plan modifications in response to the patient's changing needs and circumstances.

Putting Together A Support Network

Individuals with CAD should not go on the path to overcome it alone. Having a strong support network is essential for emotional health and long-term motivation. Family members, friends, and even support groups where people with comparable health issues can exchange experiences might all be a part of this network of support. It is important to recognize the psychological effects of CAD, and having a solid support system can help reduce stress and promote optimism. Healthcare professionals should promote a collaborative approach outside of the clinical setting by encouraging patients to include their support network in the management plan. Moreover, offering resources for mental health support or counseling can improve the general wellbeing of people attempting to recover from CAD.

In conclusion, treating coronary artery disease is a complex process that goes beyond prescription treatments. A comprehensive grasp of the diagnosis, realistic goal-setting, medication adherence, health monitoring, efficient communication with healthcare providers, and the development of a strong support system are all essential components of patient education and empowerment during this journey.

Through a holistic approach that customises tactics to meet the unique needs of each patient, healthcare providers can empower and educate their patients, improving the efficacy of CAD management and leading to better cardiovascular outcomes.

CHAPTER SIX
PREVENTING CORONARY ARTERY DISEASE

Primary and secondary prevention measures are part of a complex strategy to avoid coronary artery disease. The goal of these tactics is to lessen the prevalence and severity of coronary artery disease (CAD), which is the world's largest cause of morbidity and death. In terms of primary prevention, people can reduce risk factors linked to CAD by implementing healthy lifestyle choices. This entails using alcohol in moderation, abstaining from tobacco, exercising frequently, and maintaining a balanced diet.

Making healthy lifestyle choices is crucial for CAD primary prevention. Through the control of blood pressure, body weight, and cholesterol levels, a diet rich in fruits, vegetables, whole grains, and lean proteins that is well-balanced promotes overall cardiovascular health.

Another pillar is regular exercise, which strengthens heart function, increases blood circulation, and helps maintain ideal body weight. Since smoking is a substantial risk factor for the development of atherosclerosis and subsequent coronary events, abstaining from tobacco use is imperative given its direct link to CAD. In a similar vein, it is advisable to moderate alcohol intake because too much of it might raise blood pressure and hasten the onset of CAD.

An further crucial component of primary prevention is screening and early detection. Early risk factor identification is made possible by routine blood pressure checks, cholesterol screenings, and health examinations. Targeted therapies can be implemented to minimize these risk factors and stop the progression of CAD when CAD is detected early. Screening can also reveal genetic predispositions, allowing for the individualized prevention of those who are more vulnerable.

Now for secondary preventive measures: for those who have already had a cardiac event, cardiac rehabilitation is essential to their recovery and to preventing future episodes. This all-inclusive program includes counseling to address the psychological effects of a cardiac episode, instruction on heart-healthy living, and supervised exercise. In cardiac rehabilitation programs, exercise training lowers blood pressure, increases cardiovascular fitness, and improves general wellbeing. The teaching component encourages people to take an active role in their heart health by focusing on stress management, medication adherence, and lifestyle changes.

Since long-term management include consistent efforts to reduce risk factors and stop cardiac episodes from happening again, it is crucial for the secondary prevention of CAD. Patients may be administered antiplatelet agents to prevent blood clot formation, statins to lower cholesterol levels, and antihypertensive meds to control blood pressure. Adherence to medication is crucial. For long-term benefit, lifestyle adjustments made during cardiac rehabilitation, such as eating adjustments and frequent exercise, should be maintained. Following up with medical professionals on a regular basis guarantees continuous monitoring and treatment plan modifications based on patient requirements and responses.

primary and secondary prevention techniques must be used in tandem with a thorough and ongoing effort to avoid coronary artery disease. Primary prevention is based on healthy lifestyle choices and early diagnosis through screening; for those who have already had a cardiac event, secondary prevention interventions, such as cardiac rehabilitation and long-term care, are critical. A heart-healthy lifestyle and the management of modifiable risk factors can help people greatly lower their risk of developing CAD and enhance their general cardiovascular health.

CHAPTER SEVEN
INTEGRATIVE STRATEGIES FOR HOLISTIC HEART HEALTH

Coronary artery disease (CAD) is still a major worldwide health concern that requires a multifaceted strategy that goes beyond traditional medical treatments. Integrative methods, which highlight the relationship between the body and mind, are becoming more and more popular as effective means of advancing heart health in its whole. These methods acknowledge the complex interactions of behavioral, psychological, and physiological aspects in the onset and course of CAD.

1. Body-Mind Exercises

Integrative methods of treating coronary artery disease are based on mind-body techniques. Particularly in relation to their potential advantages in reducing stress—a known risk factor for CAD—

meditation and mindfulness practices have drawn interest. Concentrated attention and deliberate breathing are key components of meditation, which encourages relaxation and lowers the activity of the sympathetic nervous system. Conversely, mindfulness promotes judgment-free awareness of the present moment, which has a beneficial effect on psychological well-being and may have an impact on cardiovascular health.

Within the mind-body paradigm, yoga, an age-old Indian practice, has gained popularity as a holistic approach to heart health. Yoga addresses stress and improves cardiovascular function by using breath control and meditation in addition to its physical postures. Studies indicate that consistent yoga practice may help to lower blood pressure, enhance heart rate variability, and improve endothelial function, all of which may help to prevent and treat coronary artery disease (CAD).

2. Adjunctive Therapies

When combined with traditional medical treatments, complementary therapies include a wide range of practices that are intended to improve general health. The possible cardiovascular advantages of herbal supplements like garlic, hawthorn, and omega-3 fatty acids have been studied. These supplements offer an additional treatment option for CAD by potentially influencing blood pressure, inflammation, and lipid profiles. Nonetheless, it is imperative to carefully evaluate any possible interactions with prescribed drugs, underscoring the significance of an integrated and well-coordinated approach to treatment.

In acupuncture, tiny needles are inserted into predetermined body sites in accordance with traditional Chinese medical protocol. Promising findings from studies investigating the effects of acupuncture on cardiovascular health include enhanced blood flow, decreased inflammation, and autonomic nervous system modulation. A holistic approach to resolving underlying imbalances, acupuncture has potential as a supplementary therapy in the management of CAD, while more research is necessary.

3. Using Holistic Methods in addition to Medical Treatment

Integrative methods for treating coronary artery disease should be considered a supplement to traditional medical treatments, not as a replacement for them. The goal of holistic approaches is to work in concert with medical treatments, surgery, and lifestyle changes. A comprehensive and customized approach to treating CAD is ensured by developing a single treatment plan that combines integrative and conventional components.

More subtle and individualized approaches to CAD are made possible by the incorporation of complementary therapies and mind-body activities into traditional medical frameworks. In addition to traditional treatments such as antiplatelet medicines, statins, and revascularization operations, holistic therapy can address the complex character of the disease. Because physical and mental health are intertwined, this integrative paradigm emphasizes the value of treating the patient as a whole.

overcoming coronary artery disease necessitates a multimodal strategy that cuts over conventional medical lines. When combined with medical treatment, integrative approaches—which include mind-body practices, complementary therapies, and holistic strategies—offer a potential way to address the complicated character of CAD. Healthcare professionals can offer more thorough and individualized interventions by acknowledging the connection between physiological and psychological aspects, eventually supporting holistic heart health. The field of integrative cardiology is constantly changing, which emphasizes the importance of further study and cooperation between traditional and alternative medicine to improve patient outcomes in the face of this common cardiovascular issue.

CHAPTER EIGHT
OVERCOMING DIFFICULTIES AND ADAPTING TO CHANGE

Coronary artery disease (CAD) is a complex condition that requires adjustments to lifestyle and emotions in addition to its physiological effects. In order to effectively treat CAD, one must address all of its manifestations, paying special attention to emotional health and making the required lifestyle changes. This all-encompassing strategy seeks to improve the general quality of life for CAD patients in addition to managing the condition.

Handling the Psychological Impact of Coronary Artery Disease

Dealing with a variety of emotional difficulties is part of having coronary artery disease, and these difficulties can have a serious effect on one's mental well-being. Patients with CAD frequently experience anxiety and depression, which is frequently brought on by awareness of their illness and the possible restrictions it may place on their lives. These mental health problems are made worse by the persistent threat of cardiovascular events and the requirement for continuous medical management, which raise stress levels. In order to manage CAD holistically, it is essential to address depression and anxiety. This calls for a combination of pharmaceutical interventions, psychotherapy, and support groups.

The Fear of Recurrence is a roughly related emotional challenge. After a cardiac incident, people frequently suffer from a persistent worry of relapsing. This anxiety may raise stress levels, which may result in more cardiac episodes.

The development of coping strategies and psychological therapies is essential in order to reduce the anxiety of recurrence and enable patients to concentrate on their general health and preventative measures.

Handling Changes In Lifestyle

Significant lifestyle changes are required for CAD in order to control risk factors and improve cardiovascular health in general. These modifications could involve giving up smoking, starting a regular exercise regimen, and eating a heart-healthy diet. These changes are difficult to implement and call for a multifaceted strategy. Education is essential for enabling people to comprehend the reasoning for these changes and take an active role in their own well-being. It is imperative for health practitioners to offer tailored advice that considers cultural and personal preferences in order to guarantee sustained compliance with these lifestyle changes.

Managing Relationship and Social Dynamics

Beyond the person, CAD has an impact on relationships and society dynamics. Emotional strain can also be experienced by friends, family, and partners who help their loved ones deal with the difficulties of having a chronic illness. Navigating these interactions requires open and honest communication, which promotes understanding and support. Social networks and support groups, which link others going through similar things and foster a sense of community, can be very helpful resources. It is critical to address the psychosocial components of CAD in the larger framework of interpersonal connections as well as at the individual level.

In summary, overcoming coronary artery disease necessitates a comprehensive strategy that extends beyond pharmaceutical treatments.

A holistic approach must acknowledge and handle the emotional aspects of CAD, effectively manage lifestyle adjustments, and navigate social and relationship problems. Healthcare providers can enable patients affected by CAD to lead fulfilling lives and manage their illness by acknowledging the interconnectivity of these aspects. This strategy strengthens the resilience of the larger support system that surrounds the person in addition to improving their own well-being.

CHAPTER NINE
INSPIRATIONAL TALES AND TESTIMONIALS

A multidisciplinary strategy that combines lifestyle modifications and medication therapies is frequently used to treat coronary artery disease (CAD). Testimonials and inspirational stories are essential in inspiring people to take on the difficult task of conquering CAD. These stories, which are frequently told by survivors, offer a unique perspective on the hardships, victories, and life-altering events that are actually connected to the illness.

The human side of managing coronary artery disease is shown in Real-Life Journeys of Conquering Coronary Artery Disease.

These narratives usually describe the first diagnosis, the ensuing emotional turmoil, and the ensuing attempts to recover control over one's health. People who are struggling with CAD can get comfort and assurance from these stories that they are not traveling alone. The personal accounts illuminate the many tactics utilized by those who have survived, which encompass medical procedures such as bypass surgery and angioplasty in addition to adopting more health-conscious lifestyles.

Encouraging Narratives of Lifestyle Metamorphosis highlight the importance of behavioral adjustments in the treatment of CAD. In these narratives, lifestyle changes including dietary alterations, regular exercise, stress management, and quitting smoking are often emphasized. People talk about how adopting healthier lifestyle choices—often under the direction of medical professionals—improved their cardiovascular health significantly.

These tales offer hope because they show how adopting healthier lifestyle choices may be life-changing and essential for managing CAD and preventing its recurrence.

The mental health of CAD sufferers is improved by these motivational tales. Overcoming CAD is a difficult road filled with uncertainty, dread, and anxiety. But through these stories, people might find courage in the tenacity of those who have experienced similar things.

These narratives also help CAD patients feel more connected to one another by promoting a network of support where experiences are shared, counsel is given, and emotional support is easily accessible.

Examining these accounts in an academic setting can offer insightful information on the psychological components of managing CAD. It makes it possible for academics and medical professionals to comprehend the difficulties that patients encounter personally, which promotes the creation of more comprehensive and patient-centered CAD care strategies.

Medical experts can customize interventions that not only address the physiological components of CAD but also address the mental and emotional well-being of their patients by understanding the emotional and psychological dimensions of the condition.

CONCLUSION

the treatment of Coronary Artery Disease (CAD) is a dynamic and intricate process that requires a thorough comprehension of the lifestyle and medical aspects involved. Testimonials and inspirational tales are effective resources in this effort because they provide firsthand experiences of people who have overcome CAD. In addition to highlighting the wide range of medical procedures and therapy techniques used by survivors,

The Real-Life Journeys of Conquering Coronary Artery Disease also demonstrate the tenacity and resolve needed in the face of this difficult health problem.

Furthermore, the importance of lifestyle changes in CAD management is emphasized in Empowering Stories of Lifestyle Transformation.

These stories highlight how crucial healthy eating habits, consistent exercise, managing stress, and giving up smoking are for maintaining cardiovascular health.

Through sharing their stories, people not only reveal the physical improvements brought about by these lifestyle adjustments, but also the significant effects they have on their general wellbeing.

Examining these stories from an academic standpoint offers insightful information on the psychological aspects of CAD.

Developing more patient-centric healthcare practices is made possible by an understanding of the psychological and emotional elements of the illness. Empathetic and comprehensive care for patients with CAD can be improved by incorporating the lessons from these tales into medical education and practice.

Ultimately, the quest to overcome coronary artery disease is not just a medical achievement but also a profound investigation into the resiliency and transformative potential of the human spirit. We obtain a thorough understanding of CAD and open the door to a more caring and efficient method of managing and preventing it by combining the medical and personal narratives.